TYPE 2 DIABETES INSTANT POT COOKBOOK

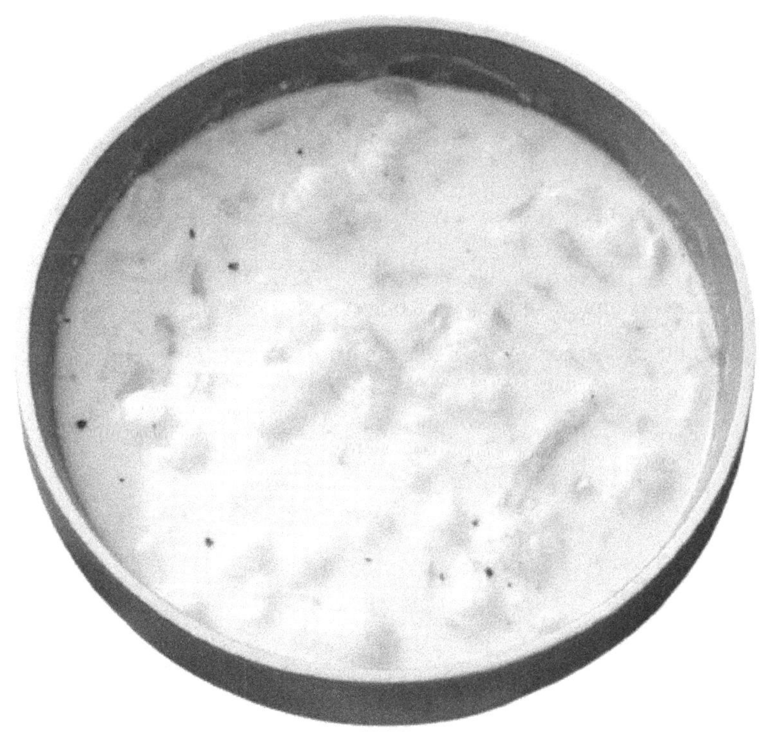

LORENE PEACHEY

DISCLAIMER

The content within this book reflects my thoughts, experiences, and beliefs. It is meant for informational and entertainment purposes. While I have taken great care to provide accurate information, I cannot guarantee the absolute correctness or applicability of the content to every individual or situation. Please consult with relevant professionals for advice specific to your needs.

TABLE OF CONTENTS

INTRODUCTION

Hello, dear reader! I am Nutrionist Lorene Peachey, and I invite you to embark on a delightful and life-changing culinary adventure with me. Picture this: a world filled with scrumptious, satisfying meals that not only tantalize your taste buds but also empower you in your journey to manage Type 2 Diabetes. Welcome to my kitchen, where the magic happens, and where I have witnessed firsthand the transformative power of my recipes.

Allow me to share a heartwarming story with you. Meet Alice Thornton, a spirited soul with a penchant for flavourful dishes and an indomitable spirit. Alice, like many, found herself navigating the labyrinth of Type 2 Diabetes, searching for a way to Savor delicious meals without compromising her health. She had tried numerous cookbooks, each promising a path to culinary delight and well-being, but alas, they left her wanting.

One fateful day, Alice stumbled upon my cookbook "Type 2 Diabetes Instant Pot Cookbook." Little did she know that this culinary compendium would be the catalyst for a transformative journey. Alice had encountered recipes before, but none resonated quite like these. The Flavors were vibrant, the ingredients easily accessible, and the preparation surprisingly effortless with the trusty Instant Pot.

As I received Alice's heartfelt letter, a symphony of emotions played within me. She spoke of the joy of savouring meals that felt like a warm hug for her taste buds, coupled with the assurance that each dish adhered to her dietary needs. The frustration of failed attempts with other cookbooks transformed into a dance of triumph, and Alice revelled in newfound culinary bliss.

I could sense Alice's gratitude through her words, as the recipes became more than just a collection of instructions—they became a lifeline, a source of comfort, and a beacon of hope. Her blood sugar levels stabilized, energy levels soared, and the seemingly daunting journey of managing diabetes took on a brighter hue.

Now, let's dive into the core of why embracing healthy diabetes-friendly foods is not just a culinary choice but a transformative lifestyle decision. Imagine the benefits of indulging in meals that are not only palatable but also nourish your body from within. What if every bite you took contributed to better blood sugar control, enhanced energy levels, and a shield against the complications that often accompany Type 2 Diabetes?

Eating healthy is not a mere checkbox on a to-do list; it's a commitment to your well-being. It's about questioning the consequences of consuming foods laden with sugars, unhealthy fats, and processed ingredients. How many times have we succumbed to the allure of a sweet treat only to find ourselves on a rollercoaster of energy crashes and sugar spikes?

Consider this: what if each meal you prepared and enjoyed was a step towards a healthier, more vibrant you? What if the act of cooking became a form of self-love, a ritual of nourishment that extended beyond the kitchen into every facet of your life? The dangers of unhealthy eating are not just numbers on a nutritional label; they manifest as fatigue, mood swings, and, in the long run, potential complications that could alter the course of your life.

Now, let's shift our focus to the advantages and unparalleled benefits of having my cookbook, "Type 2 Diabetes Instant Pot Cookbook," as your culinary companion. Picture a world where meal preparation is a joy rather than a chore. Imagine the thrill of serving up dishes that not only satisfy your cravings but also contribute to your overall health.

This cookbook is not merely a collection of recipes; it's a handbook for empowerment. The Instant Pot, your kitchen ally, transforms the way you approach cooking, making it efficient, convenient, and, above all, enjoyable. My recipes are crafted with precision, ensuring a harmonious blend of Flavors while keeping a watchful eye on your blood sugar levels.

As you peruse the pages of this cookbook, envision the freedom of exploring diverse cuisines without the fear of compromising your health. From breakfast delights to hearty main courses, flavourful side dishes, and indulgent desserts, each recipe is a testament to the notion that eating for wellness can be an exhilarating journey.

And now, dear reader, I extend an invitation. An invitation to join me on this culinary expedition where each dish is a celebration of life and health. Let's embrace the joy of savouring meals that nourish not just our bodies but our souls. Let the journey begin, and may each recipe be a stepping stone towards a healthier, happier you.

So, shall we venture into the realm of Instant Pot magic together? Open the book, let the aroma of wholesome goodness waft through your kitchen, and let's make each meal a testimony to the vibrant, flavourful life that awaits you.

Contact the Author

Thank you for reading my book! I would love to hear from you, whether you have feedback, questions, or just want to share your thoughts. Your feedback means a lot to me and helps me improve as a writer.

Please don't hesitate to reach out to me through

lorenepeachey@gmail.com

I look forward to connecting with my readers and appreciate your support in this literary journey. Your thoughts and comments are valuable to me.

CHAPTER 1

UNDERSTANDING TYPE 2 DIABETES

Type 2 diabetes is a chronic condition that affects the way your body metabolizes sugar (glucose), an important source of fuel for the body. In individuals with type 2 diabetes, the body either resists the effects of insulin – a hormone that regulates the movement of sugar into your cells – or doesn't produce enough insulin to maintain normal glucose levels.

There are several risk factors for developing type 2 diabetes, including genetics, age, obesity, and lack of physical activity. The condition can lead to various complications such as heart disease, stroke, kidney disease, and nerve damage if not managed effectively.

Managing type 2 diabetes involves making lifestyle changes, including a balanced diet, regular exercise, and medication if necessary. Monitoring blood sugar levels is crucial for keeping the condition under control. It's also important to be aware of the glycemic index of foods, which indicates how quickly a particular food can raise blood sugar levels.

Benefits of Using an Instant Pot for Diabetes-friendly Cooking:

The Instant Pot, a versatile electric pressure cooker, can be a valuable tool for individuals managing type 2 diabetes. Here are some benefits of using an Instant Pot for diabetes-friendly cooking:

Time Efficiency: The Instant Pot significantly reduces cooking time, making it convenient for individuals with busy schedules. Quick cooking helps preserve the nutritional content of food and can encourage the consumption of freshly prepared meals.

Preservation of Nutrients: The sealed environment of the Instant Pot helps retain more vitamins and minerals in food compared to traditional cooking methods. This is particularly important for individuals with diabetes, as a nutrient-rich diet plays a crucial role in overall health.

Portion Control: The Instant Pot allows for precise portion control, helping individuals manage their carbohydrate intake, which is a key consideration for those with diabetes. This can assist in regulating blood sugar levels and promoting **better overall health.**

One-Pot Meals: The Instant Pot is ideal for preparing one-pot meals, minimizing the need for added fats and oils. This can contribute to weight management, an important aspect of diabetes care, as excess weight can exacerbate insulin resistance.

Versatility in Cooking: The Instant Pot can be used for a variety of cooking methods, including steaming, sautéing, and slow cooking. This versatility allows for the preparation of a wide range of diabetes-friendly recipes, from soups and stews to lean protein and vegetable dishes.

Enhanced Flavor: The sealed cooking environment in the Instant Pot helps flavors meld together, resulting in rich and savory dishes without the need for excessive salt or sugar. This is beneficial for individuals with diabetes who need to be mindful of their sodium and sugar intake.

CHAPTER 2

GETTING STARTED

Choosing the right Instant Pot for your needs is essential to make the most of this versatile kitchen appliance. Consider the following factors when selecting an Instant Pot:

Size Matters: Instant Pots come in various sizes, typically ranging from 3 to 8 quarts. Choose a size that suits the number of people you usually cook for. A 6-quart Instant Pot is a popular choice for most households.

Features: Different models of Instant Pots come with various features such as pressure cooking, slow cooking, sautéing, and more. Consider your cooking preferences and needs when selecting a model with the right features.

Budget: Instant Pots are available at different price points. While some models come with advanced features, basic models are often sufficient for everyday cooking. Determine your budget and choose accordingly.

Essential Tools and Ingredients:

To make your Instant Pot cooking experience smooth and enjoyable, gather the following tools and ingredients:

Tools:

Instant Pot Accessories: Invest in additional accessories like a steamer basket, trivet, and silicone sealing rings to expand your Instant Pot's capabilities.

Kitchen Scale: Precise measurements are crucial in cooking, especially for individuals managing diabetes. A kitchen scale helps you measure ingredients accurately.

Wooden or Silicone Utensils: Use non-metallic utensils to avoid damaging the Instant Pot's non-stick coating.

Cutting Board and Sharp Knife: Essential tools for preparing ingredients before cooking.

Ingredients:

Low-Glycemic Carbohydrates: Opt for whole grains, legumes, and vegetables with a low glycemic index to help manage blood sugar levels.

Lean Proteins: Include sources of lean protein such as chicken, turkey, fish, tofu, and legumes in your recipes.

Healthy Fats: Use heart-healthy fats like olive oil, avocados, and nuts in moderation.

Fresh Herbs and Spices: Enhance flavor without relying on excessive salt or sugar by using fresh herbs and a variety of spices.

Broths and Low-Sodium Sauces: Flavor your dishes with low-sodium broths and sauces to add depth without compromising on health.

Tips for Safe and Efficient Instant Pot Cooking:

Read the Manual: Familiarize yourself with the Instant Pot manual to understand its features, functions, and safety guidelines.

Use Proper Sealing: Ensure the Instant Pot is properly sealed before cooking under pressure. This is crucial for the appliance to work effectively.

Allow for Natural Pressure Release: For certain recipes, allowing the Instant Pot to release pressure naturally can enhance the texture and flavor of your dishes.

Adjust Cooking Times: As you become more familiar with your Instant Pot, you can adjust cooking times to suit your preferences and ensure optimal results.

Experiment with Recipes: The Instant Pot is incredibly versatile. Experiment with different recipes to discover the full range of dishes you can prepare with this appliance.

Clean your Instant Pot regularly, including the sealing ring and steam release valve, to prevent any issues and ensure longevity.

CHAPTER 3

BREAKFAST DELIGHTS

Quinoa Breakfast Bowl

Cooking Time: 10 minutes

Serving: 2

Ingredients:

- ✓ 1 cup quinoa
- ✓ 2 cups almond milk
- ✓ 1 teaspoon cinnamon
- ✓ 1/2 cup berries
- ✓ 1 tablespoon chopped nuts.

Instructions:

1. Rinse quinoa and combine with almond milk and cinnamon in the Instant Pot.
2. Cook on high pressure for 1 minute, then natural release.
3. Serve topped with berries and nuts.

Nutritional Information: 300 calories, 45g carbs, 10g protein, 8g fat, 6g fiber

This protein-packed breakfast stabilizes blood sugar levels.

Egg Muffins with Spinach and Feta

Cooking Time: 8 minutes

Serving: 4

Ingredients:

- ✓ 6 eggs
- ✓ 1 cup fresh spinach
- ✓ 1/2 cup feta cheese
- ✓ Salt and pepper to taste
- ✓ Cooking spray

Instructions:

1. Whisk eggs and season with salt and pepper.
2. Stir in spinach and feta.
3. Pour mixture into greased silicone muffin cups.
4. Cook on high pressure for 8 minutes.

Nutritional Information: 180 calories, 2g carbs, 14g protein, 12g fat, 1g fiber

Packed with protein, these muffins are a convenient and low-carb breakfast option.

Oatmeal with Apples and Cinnamon

Cooking Time: 4 minutes

Serving: 3

Ingredients:

- ✓ 1 cup steel-cut oats
- ✓ 2 apples, diced.
- ✓ 1 teaspoon cinnamon
- ✓ 2 tablespoons maple syrup
- ✓ 2 1/2 cups water

Instructions:

1. Combine oats, apples, cinnamon, maple syrup, and water in the Instant Pot.
2. Cook on high pressure for 4 minutes, then quick release.

Nutritional Information: 250 calories, 50g carbs, 5g protein, 3g fat, 7g fiber

A fiber-rich breakfast to keep you full and satisfied.

Greek Yogurt Parfait

Cooking Time: 1 minute (for pressure cooking grains)

Serving: 2

Ingredients:

- ✓ 1 cup Greek yogurt
- ✓ 1/2 cup granola (preferably low sugar)
- ✓ 1/2 cup mixed berries
- ✓ 1 tablespoon honey

Instructions:

1. Layer Greek yogurt, granola, and berries in jars.
2. Drizzle honey on top.
3. Pressure cook grains separately for added texture.

Nutritional Information: 280 calories, 30g carbs, 15g protein, 10g fat, 4g fiber

A quick and delightful parfait with a balance of protein and carbs.

Sweet Potato Breakfast Hash

Cooking Time: 15 minutes

Serving: 4

Ingredients:

- ✓ 2 sweet potatoes, diced
- ✓ 1 bell pepper, diced
- ✓ 1 onion, chopped
- ✓ 1 teaspoon paprika
- ✓ 1/2 teaspoon garlic powder

Instructions:

1. Toss sweet potatoes, bell pepper, and onion in the Instant Pot.
2. Add paprika and garlic powder.
3. Cook on high pressure for 5 minutes.

Nutritional Information: 220 calories, 45g carbs, 4g protein, 2g fat, 8g fiber

A nutrient-dense, veggie-packed hash for a savory breakfast.

Chia Seed Pudding

Cooking Time: 5 minutes (plus chilling time)

Serving: 3

Ingredients:

- ✓ 1/2 cup chia seeds
- ✓ 2 cups almond milk
- ✓ 1 teaspoon vanilla extract
- ✓ 2 tablespoons sugar-free sweetener
- ✓ Fresh berries for topping

Instructions:

1. Mix chia seeds, almond milk, vanilla extract, and sweetener in the Instant Pot.
2. Cook on sauté mode for 5 minutes, stirring continuously.
3. Chill in the refrigerator before serving with berries.

Nutritional Information: 150 calories, 15g carbs, 5g protein, 8g fat, 10g fiber

Chia seeds provide omega-3 fatty acids and fiber for a nutritious breakfast.

Turkey Sausage and Vegetable Frittata

Cooking Time: 10 minutes

Serving: 6

Ingredients:

- ✓ 8 eggs
- ✓ 1/2 cup milk
- ✓ 1 cup turkey sausage, cooked and crumbled
- ✓ 1 cup mixed vegetables (bell peppers, spinach, tomatoes)
- ✓ Salt and pepper to taste

Instructions:

1. Whisk eggs, milk, salt, and pepper.
2. Stir in cooked turkey sausage and vegetables.
3. Pour mixture into a greased Instant Pot.
4. Cook on high pressure for 8 minutes.

Nutritional Information: 220 calories, 5g carbs, 15g protein, 15g fat, 2g fiber

A protein-packed frittata with lean turkey sausage and colorful veggies.

Cauliflower "Rice" Breakfast Bowl

Cooking Time: 5 minutes

Serving: 4

Ingredients:

- ✓ 1 head cauliflower, grated
- ✓ 1 cup diced ham
- ✓ 1/2 cup green onions, chopped
- ✓ 2 eggs, beaten
- ✓ 1 tablespoon soy sauce (low-sodium)

Instructions:

1. Sauté cauliflower, ham, and green onions in the Instant Pot.
2. Push ingredients to the side, pour beaten eggs, and scramble.
3. Stir in soy sauce.

Nutritional Information: 180 calories, 10g carbs, 15g protein, 8g fat, 4g fiber

A low-carb, savory breakfast bowl with the goodness of cauliflower.

Blueberry Almond Steel-Cut Oats

Cooking Time: 10 minutes

Serving: 4

Ingredients:

- ✓ 1 cup steel-cut oats
- ✓ 1 cup fresh blueberries
- ✓ 1/2 cup sliced almonds
- ✓ 1 teaspoon vanilla extract
- ✓ 3 cups water

Instructions:

1. Combine oats, blueberries, almonds, vanilla, and water in the Instant Pot.
2. Cook on high pressure for 6 minutes, then natural release.

Nutritional Information: 230 calories, 30g carbs, 7g protein, 10g fat, 6g fiber

Antioxidant-rich blueberries and almonds add flavor and nutrients to this oatmeal.

Mushroom and Spinach Breakfast Risotto

Cooking Time: 12 minutes

Serving: 4

Ingredients:

- ✓ 1 cup Arborio rice
- ✓ 1 cup mushrooms, sliced
- ✓ 2 cups fresh spinach
- ✓ 1 onion, finely chopped
- ✓ 4 cups vegetable broth
- ✓ 1/4 cup Parmesan cheese (optional)

Instructions:

1. Sauté mushrooms and onions in the Instant Pot.
2. Add Arborio rice and stir.
3. Pour in vegetable broth and cook on high pressure for 8 minutes.
4. Stir in fresh spinach and, if desired, Parmesan cheese.

Nutritional Information: 280 calories, 45g carbs, 6g protein, 7g fat, 5g fiber

A savory and satisfying breakfast risotto with a mix of veggies

CHAPTER 4

SATISFYING SOUPS

Vegetable and Lentil Soup

Cooking Time: 15 minutes

Serving: 6

Ingredients:

- ✓ 1 cup green lentils
- ✓ 4 cups mixed vegetables (carrots, celery, zucchini)
- ✓ 1 onion, diced
- ✓ 4 cups low-sodium vegetable broth
- ✓ 1 teaspoon cumin
- ✓ Salt and pepper to taste

Instructions:

1. Combine all ingredients in the Instant Pot.
2. Cook on high pressure for 10 minutes.
3. Season with cumin, salt, and pepper.

Nutritional Information: 200 calories, 35g carbs, 12g protein, 1g fat, 8g fiber

A hearty, fiber-rich soup that aids in blood sugar control.

Chicken and Quinoa Soup

Cooking Time: 20 minutes

Serving: 4

Ingredients:

- ✓ 1 lb boneless, skinless chicken breasts
- ✓ 1/2 cup quinoa
- ✓ 4 cups low-sodium chicken broth
- ✓ 2 carrots, sliced
- ✓ 2 celery stalks, chopped
- ✓ 1 teaspoon thyme

Instructions:

1. Place all ingredients in the Instant Pot.
2. Cook on high pressure for 15 minutes.
3. Shred chicken before serving.

Nutritional Information: 250 calories, 20g carbs, 25g protein, 6g fat, 3g fiber

Protein-packed with quinoa, this soup is a balanced meal option.

Spinach and Mushroom Egg Drop Soup

Cooking Time: 8 minutes

Serving: 4

Ingredients:

- ✓ 4 cups low-sodium chicken broth
- ✓ 2 cups spinach
- ✓ 1 cup mushrooms, sliced
- ✓ 2 eggs, beaten
- ✓ 1 teaspoon ginger, minced
- ✓ Soy sauce to taste

Instructions:

1. Bring chicken broth, ginger, and soy sauce to a simmer in the Instant Pot.
2. Add mushrooms and spinach.
3. Slowly pour beaten eggs into the soup, stirring gently.

Nutritional Information: 120 calories, 10g carbs, 10g protein, 5g fat, 3g fiber

A low-calorie, nutrient-dense soup with the richness of eggs and earthy mushrooms.

Turmeric Cauliflower Soup

Cooking Time: 12 minutes

Serving: 4

Ingredients:

- ✓ 1 head cauliflower, chopped
- ✓ 1 onion, diced
- ✓ 2 teaspoons turmeric
- ✓ 4 cups vegetable broth
- ✓ 1 can coconut milk (light)
- ✓ Salt and pepper to taste

Instructions:

1. Sauté onions and cauliflower in the Instant Pot.
2. Add turmeric, vegetable broth, and coconut milk.
3. Cook on high pressure for 8 minutes.

Nutritional Information: 180 calories, 20g carbs, 5g protein, 10g fat, 6g fiber

A warming soup with anti-inflammatory turmeric and the creaminess of coconut milk.

Salmon and Kale Chowder

Cooking Time: 15 minutes

Serving: 4

Ingredients:

- ✓ 1 lb salmon fillets, cubed
- ✓ 4 cups kale, chopped
- ✓ 1 onion, finely chopped
- ✓ 2 potatoes, diced
- ✓ 4 cups low-sodium fish broth
- ✓ 1/2 cup low-fat milk

Instructions:

1. Sauté onions and potatoes in the Instant Pot.
2. Add salmon, kale, fish broth, and milk.
3. Cook on high pressure for 10 minutes.

Nutritional Information: 280 calories, 30g carbs, 30g protein, 6g fat, 5g fiber

A protein-rich chowder with the goodness of salmon and kale.

Black Bean and Turkey Chili

Cooking Time: 25 minutes

Serving: 6

Ingredients:

- ✓ 1 lb ground turkey
- ✓ 2 cans black beans, drained and rinsed
- ✓ 1 can diced tomatoes
- ✓ 1 onion, diced
- ✓ 2 teaspoons chili powder
- ✓ 4 cups low-sodium chicken broth

Instructions:

1. Brown turkey and onions in the Instant Pot.
2. Add beans, tomatoes, chili powder, and chicken broth.
3. Cook on high pressure for 15 minutes.

Nutritional Information: 240 calories, 30g carbs, 25g protein, 5g fat, 10g fiber

A protein-packed chili with fiber-rich black beans for stable blood sugar.

Miso Soup with Tofu and Seaweed

Cooking Time: 10 minutes

Serving: 4

Ingredients:

- ✓ 4 cups low-sodium vegetable broth
- ✓ 1/2 cup miso paste
- ✓ 1 cup tofu, cubed
- ✓ 2 sheets seaweed, shredded
- ✓ Green onions for garnish

Instructions:

1. Whisk miso paste into vegetable broth in the Instant Pot.
2. Add tofu and seaweed.
3. Cook on high pressure for 5 minutes.

Nutritional Information: 150 calories, 15g carbs, 10g protein, 8g fat, 3g fiber

A low-calorie, savory soup with the umami flavor of miso and the goodness of tofu.

Cabbage and Sausage Soup

Cooking Time: 12 minutes

Serving: 6

Ingredients:

- ✓ 1/2 head cabbage, shredded
- ✓ 1 lb turkey sausage, sliced
- ✓ 1 onion, chopped
- ✓ 2 carrots, sliced
- ✓ 4 cups low-sodium chicken broth
- ✓ 1 teaspoon Italian seasoning

Instructions:

1. Sauté sausage, onions, and carrots in the Instant Pot.
2. Add cabbage, chicken broth, and Italian seasoning.
3. Cook on high pressure for 8 minutes.

Nutritional Information: 220 calories, 15g carbs, 15g protein, 10g fat, 5g fiber

A low-carb, flavorful soup with lean turkey sausage and plenty of veggies.

Butternut Squash and Apple Soup

Cooking Time: 15 minutes

Serving: 4

Ingredients:

- ✓ 1 butternut squash, peeled and cubed
- ✓ 2 apples, peeled and chopped
- ✓ 1 onion, diced
- ✓ 4 cups low-sodium vegetable broth
- ✓ 1 teaspoon cinnamon
- ✓ Salt and pepper to taste

Instructions:

1. Combine squash, apples, onions, and vegetable broth in the Instant Pot.
2. Cook on high pressure for 10 minutes.
3. Purée the soup, add cinnamon, salt, and pepper.

Nutritional Information: 180 calories, 40g carbs, 3g protein, 1g fat, 6g fiber

A sweet and savory soup loaded with vitamins and antioxidants.

Shrimp and Vegetable Gumbo

Cooking Time: 20 minutes

Serving: 4

Ingredients:

- ✓ 1 lb shrimp, peeled and deveined
- ✓ 1 bell pepper, chopped
- ✓ 1 onion, diced
- ✓ 2 celery stalks, sliced
- ✓ 2 tomatoes, diced
- ✓ 4 cups low-sodium chicken broth
- ✓ 1 tablespoon Cajun seasoning

Instructions:

1. Sauté shrimp, onions, peppers, and celery in the Instant Pot.
2. Add tomatoes, chicken broth, and Cajun seasoning.
3. Cook on high pressure for 15 minutes.

Nutritional Information: 250 calories, 15g carbs, 30g protein, 6g fat, 3g fiber

A spicy and protein-rich gumbo with a mix of colorful vegetables.

CHAPTER 5

WHOLESOME MAIN DISHES

Balsamic Chicken with Vegetables

Cooking Time: 15 minutes

Serving: 4

Ingredients:

- ✓ 1.5 lbs boneless, skinless chicken breasts
- ✓ 1 cup cherry tomatoes
- ✓ 1 bell pepper, sliced
- ✓ 1/4 cup balsamic vinegar
- ✓ 2 tablespoons olive oil
- ✓ 1 teaspoon Italian seasoning

Instructions:

1. Season chicken with salt, pepper, and Italian seasoning.
2. Sauté chicken in olive oil in the Instant Pot.
3. Add tomatoes, bell pepper, and balsamic vinegar.
4. Cook on high pressure for 8 minutes.

Nutritional Information: 280 calories, 10g carbs, 35g protein, 12g fat, 3g fiber

A flavorful, low-carb dish featuring lean protein and colorful vegetables.

Lemon Herb Salmon

Cooking Time: 5 minutes

Serving: 2

Ingredients:

- ✓ 2 salmon fillets
- ✓ 1 lemon, sliced
- ✓ 2 tablespoons fresh dill
- ✓ 1 tablespoon olive oil
- ✓ Salt and pepper to taste

Instructions:

1. Season salmon with salt and pepper.
2. Place salmon in Instant Pot, top with lemon slices and dill.
3. Drizzle with olive oil.
4. Cook on high pressure for 3 minutes.

Nutritional Information: 250 calories, 2g carbs, 30g protein, 14g fat, 1g fiber

A quick and light salmon dish rich in omega-3 fatty acids.

Turkey and Vegetable Quinoa Bowl

Cooking Time: 10 minutes

Serving: 4

Ingredients:

- ✓ 1 lb ground turkey
- ✓ 1 cup quinoa
- ✓ 2 cups mixed vegetables (broccoli, bell peppers, carrots)
- ✓ 1 can diced tomatoes
- ✓ 1 teaspoon cumin
- ✓ 1 teaspoon garlic powder

Instructions:

1. Sauté ground turkey in the Instant Pot.
2. Add quinoa, mixed vegetables, diced tomatoes, cumin, and garlic powder.
3. Cook on high pressure for 5 minutes.

Nutritional Information: 320 calories, 30g carbs, 25g protein, 12g fat, 5g fiber

A balanced bowl with lean turkey, quinoa, and a variety of colorful vegetables.

Eggplant and Chickpea Curry

Cooking Time: 15 minutes

Serving: 4

Ingredients:

- ✓ 1 large eggplant, diced
- ✓ 1 can chickpeas, drained
- ✓ 1 onion, finely chopped
- ✓ 2 tomatoes, diced
- ✓ 1/4 cup curry powder
- ✓ 1 cup vegetable broth

Instructions:

1. Sauté onions and eggplant in the Instant Pot.
2. Add chickpeas, tomatoes, curry powder, and vegetable broth.
3. Cook on high pressure for 8 minutes.

Nutritional Information: 240 calories, 40g carbs, 10g protein, 7g fat, 10g fiber

A fiber-rich curry with eggplant and chickpeas for a satisfying meal.

Garlic Herb Shrimp and Broccoli

Cooking Time: 5 minutes

Serving: 2

Ingredients:

- ✓ 1 lb shrimp, peeled and deveined
- ✓ 2 cups broccoli florets
- ✓ 4 cloves garlic, minced
- ✓ 2 tablespoons fresh parsley, chopped
- ✓ 1 tablespoon olive oil
- ✓ Lemon wedges for serving

Instructions:

1. Sauté shrimp and garlic in olive oil in the Instant Pot.
2. Add broccoli and cook on high pressure for 3 minutes.
3. Garnish with fresh parsley and serve with lemon wedges.

Nutritional Information: 220 calories, 10g carbs, 30g protein, 8g fat, 4g fiber

A quick and protein-packed dish featuring succulent shrimp and crisp broccoli.

Spaghetti Squash with Turkey Bolognese

Cooking Time: 15 minutes

Serving: 4

Ingredients:

- ✓ 1 medium spaghetti squash
- ✓ 1 lb ground turkey
- ✓ 1 can crushed tomatoes
- ✓ 1 onion, diced
- ✓ 2 cloves garlic, minced
- ✓ 1 teaspoon oregano

Instructions:

1. Cut spaghetti squash in half and remove seeds.
2. Place squash in Instant Pot, add ground turkey, tomatoes, onion, garlic, and oregano.
3. Cook on high pressure for 10 minutes.

Nutritional Information: 280 calories, 30g carbs, 25g protein, 10g fat, 8g fiber

A low-carb alternative to traditional pasta with a lean turkey bolognese.

Lentil and Vegetable Stew

Cooking Time: 12 minutes

Serving: 6

Ingredients:

- ✓ 1 cup dried lentils
- ✓ 4 cups mixed vegetables (carrots, potatoes, celery)
- ✓ 1 onion, chopped
- ✓ 4 cups vegetable broth
- ✓ 1 teaspoon thyme
- ✓ Salt and pepper to taste

Instructions:

1. Rinse lentils and place them in the Instant Pot.
2. Add mixed vegetables, onion, vegetable broth, thyme, salt, and pepper.
3. Cook on high pressure for 8 minutes.

Nutritional Information: 220 calories, 40g carbs, 15g protein, 2g fat, 10g fiber

A fiber-packed, plant-based stew that's hearty and nutritious.

Mediterranean Chicken and Quinoa Bowl

Cooking Time: 10 minutes

Serving: 4

Ingredients:

- ✓ 1.5 lbs boneless, skinless chicken thighs
- ✓ 1 cup quinoa
- ✓ 1 cup cherry tomatoes, halved
- ✓ 1 cucumber, diced
- ✓ 1/4 cup feta cheese, crumbled
- ✓ 2 tablespoons olive oil

Instructions:

1. Season chicken with salt and pepper.
2. Sauté chicken in olive oil in the Instant Pot.
3. Add quinoa, cherry tomatoes, cucumber, and feta.
4. Cook on high pressure for 5 minutes.

Nutritional Information: 320 calories, 25g carbs, 30g protein, 12g fat, 4g fiber

A Mediterranean-inspired bowl featuring lean chicken, quinoa, and fresh veggies.

Beef and Vegetable Stir-Fry

Cooking Time: 8 minutes

Serving: 4

Ingredients:

- ✓ 1 lb lean beef strips
- ✓ 2 cups broccoli florets
- ✓ 1 bell pepper, sliced
- ✓ 1 onion, thinly sliced
- ✓ 1/4 cup low-sodium soy sauce
- ✓ 1 tablespoon sesame oil

Instructions:

1. Sauté beef in sesame oil in the Instant Pot.
2. Add broccoli, bell pepper, onion, and soy sauce.
3. Cook on high pressure for 3 minutes.

Nutritional Information: 280 calories, 15g carbs, 30g protein, 12g fat, 5g fiber

A quick and flavorful stir-fry with lean beef and colorful vegetables.

Cauliflower and Chickpea Curry

Cooking Time: 12 minutes

Serving: 4

Ingredients:

- ✓ 1 head cauliflower, cut into florets
- ✓ 1 can chickpeas, drained
- ✓ 1 onion, finely chopped
- ✓ 2 tomatoes, diced
- ✓ 1/4 cup curry powder
- ✓ 1 cup vegetable broth

Instructions:

1. Sauté onions and cauliflower in the Instant Pot.
2. Add chickpeas, tomatoes, curry powder, and vegetable broth.
3. Cook on high pressure for 8 minutes.

Nutritional Information: 240 calories, 40g carbs, 10g protein, 7g fat, 10g fiber

A vegetarian curry with the heartiness of cauliflower and protein-packed chickpeas.

CHAPTER 6

FLAVORFUL SIDE DISHES

Garlic Parmesan Cauliflower Mash

Cooking Time: 10 minutes

Serving: 4

Ingredients:

- ✓ 1 head cauliflower, cut into florets
- ✓ 2 cloves garlic, minced
- ✓ 1/4 cup grated Parmesan
- ✓ 2 tablespoons butter
- ✓ Salt and pepper to taste

Instructions:

1. Steam cauliflower in Instant Pot with garlic until tender.
2. Mash with Parmesan, butter, salt, and pepper.

Nutritional Information: 120 calories, 10g carbs, 5g protein, 8g fat, 4g fiber

A low-carb alternative to mashed potatoes with the richness of garlic and Parmesan.

Lemon Herb Quinoa

Cooking Time: 5 minutes

Serving: 4

Ingredients:

- ✓ 1 cup quinoa
- ✓ 2 cups vegetable broth
- ✓ Zest and juice of 1 lemon
- ✓ 2 tablespoons chopped fresh herbs (such as parsley and thyme)
- ✓ Salt and pepper to taste

Instructions:

1. Rinse quinoa and combine with vegetable broth in Instant Pot.
2. Cook on high pressure for 1 minute.
3. Fluff with a fork and stir in lemon zest, juice, and herbs.

Nutritional Information: 180 calories, 30g carbs, 5g protein, 3g fat, 4g fiber

A light and refreshing quinoa side dish with citrusy lemon and fresh herbs.

Brussels Sprouts with Balsamic Glaze

Cooking Time: 5 minutes

Serving: 4

Ingredients:

- ✓ 1 lb Brussels sprouts, trimmed and halved
- ✓ 1/4 cup balsamic glaze
- ✓ 2 tablespoons olive oil
- ✓ Salt and pepper to taste

Instructions:

1. Toss Brussels sprouts in olive oil, salt, and pepper.
2. Sauté in Instant Pot until slightly browned.
3. Drizzle with balsamic glaze before serving.

Nutritional Information: 120 calories, 15g carbs, 4g protein, 6g fat, 4g fiber

Caramelized Brussels sprouts with a sweet and tangy balsamic glaze.

Cilantro Lime Brown Rice

Cooking Time: 12 minutes

Serving: 6

Ingredients:

- ✓ 2 cups brown rice
- ✓ 3 cups vegetable broth
- ✓ Zest and juice of 2 limes
- ✓ 1/4 cup fresh cilantro, chopped
- ✓ Salt to taste

Instructions:

1. Combine brown rice and vegetable broth in Instant Pot.
2. Cook on high pressure for 10 minutes.
3. Fluff rice and stir in lime zest, juice, and cilantro.

Nutritional Information: 200 calories, 40g carbs, 5g protein, 2g fat, 3g fiber

A zesty and flavorful brown rice side dish with the freshness of cilantro and lime.

Spiced Roasted Sweet Potatoes

Cooking Time: 10 minutes

Serving: 4

Ingredients:

- ✓ 2 sweet potatoes, peeled and cubed
- ✓ 1 teaspoon paprika
- ✓ 1 teaspoon cumin
- ✓ 2 tablespoons olive oil
- ✓ Salt and pepper to taste

Instructions:

1. Toss sweet potatoes in olive oil, paprika, cumin, salt, and pepper.
2. Roast in Instant Pot until tender and slightly crispy.

Nutritional Information: 180 calories, 25g carbs, 2g protein, 9g fat, 4g fiber

Flavorful, spiced sweet potatoes for a nutrient-rich side dish.

Tomato Basil Quinoa Salad

Cooking Time: 5 minutes

Serving: 4

Ingredients:

- ✓ 1 cup quinoa, cooked
- ✓ 1 cup cherry tomatoes, halved
- ✓ 1/4 cup fresh basil, chopped
- ✓ 2 tablespoons balsamic vinegar
- ✓ 2 tablespoons olive oil
- ✓ Salt and pepper to taste

Instructions:

1. Combine cooked quinoa, cherry tomatoes, and basil in Instant Pot.
2. Drizzle with balsamic vinegar and olive oil.
3. Season with salt and pepper.

Nutritional Information: 220 calories, 30g carbs, 5g protein, 8g fat, 4g fiber

A light and refreshing quinoa salad with the vibrant flavors of tomatoes and basil.

Sesame Ginger Green Beans

Cooking Time: 4 minutes

Serving: 4

Ingredients:

- ✓ 1 lb green beans, trimmed
- ✓ 2 tablespoons soy sauce (low-sodium)
- ✓ 1 tablespoon sesame oil
- ✓ 1 tablespoon fresh ginger, minced
- ✓ 1 tablespoon sesame seeds

Instructions:

1. Steam green beans in Instant Pot.
2. Toss with soy sauce, sesame oil, ginger, and sesame seeds.

Nutritional Information: 90 calories, 10g carbs, 3g protein, 5g fat, 4g fiber

Crunchy green beans with a savory sesame ginger glaze.

Mushroom and Spinach Quinoa Pilaf

Cooking Time: 8 minutes

Serving: 4

Ingredients:

- ✓ 1 cup quinoa
- ✓ 2 cups vegetable broth
- ✓ 1 cup mushrooms, sliced
- ✓ 2 cups fresh spinach
- ✓ 1 onion, finely chopped
- ✓ 1 tablespoon olive oil

Instructions:

1. Sauté mushrooms and onions in olive oil in Instant Pot.
2. Add quinoa, vegetable broth, and spinach.
3. Cook on high pressure for 5 minutes.

Nutritional Information: 220 calories, 30g carbs, 8g protein, 8g fat, 5g fiber

A nutrient-packed quinoa pilaf with the earthiness of mushrooms and the freshness of spinach.

Roasted Red Pepper and Feta Cauliflower Rice

Cooking Time: 5 minutes

Serving: 4

Ingredients:

- ✓ 1 head cauliflower, grated
- ✓ 1/2 cup roasted red peppers, chopped
- ✓ 1/4 cup crumbled feta cheese
- ✓ 2 tablespoons olive oil
- ✓ Salt and pepper to taste

Instructions:

1. Sauté grated cauliflower in olive oil in Instant Pot.
2. Stir in roasted red peppers and feta.
3. Season with salt and pepper.

Nutritional Information: 150 calories, 12g carbs, 6g protein, 10g fat, 5g fiber

A low-carb alternative to rice with the sweetness of roasted red peppers and the creaminess of feta.

Citrus Avocado Salad

Cooking Time: 5 minutes

Serving: 4

Ingredients:

- ✓ 2 avocados, diced
- ✓ 1 grapefruit, segmented
- ✓ 1 orange, segmented
- ✓ 1 tablespoon olive oil
- ✓ 2 tablespoons fresh mint, chopped
- ✓ Salt and pepper to taste

Instructions:

1. Combine diced avocados, grapefruit, and orange segments in Instant Pot.
2. Drizzle with olive oil, sprinkle with mint, and season with salt and pepper.

Nutritional Information: 200 calories, 15g carbs, 3g protein, 16g fat, 7g fiber

A refreshing and nutrient-rich salad with the creamy texture of avocado and the brightness of citrus.

CHAPTER 7

QUICK AND EASY SNACKS

Hummus and Veggie Dip

Cooking Time: 2 minutes (steaming in Instant Pot)

Serving: 4

Ingredients:

- ✓ 1 can chickpeas, drained
- ✓ 2 cloves garlic
- ✓ 1/4 cup tahini
- ✓ 2 tablespoons olive oil
- ✓ Assorted fresh veggies for dipping

Instructions:

1. Steam chickpeas in Instant Pot for 2 minutes.
2. Blend chickpeas, garlic, tahini, and olive oil to make hummus.
3. Serve with fresh veggie sticks.

Nutritional Information: 150 calories, 15g carbs, 5g protein, 9g fat, 6g fiber

A homemade hummus dip paired with crisp, colorful veggies for a satisfying snack.

Deviled Eggs with Avocado

Cooking Time: 5 minutes (hard-boiling eggs in Instant Pot)

Serving: 6

Ingredients:

- ✓ 6 hard-boiled eggs
- ✓ 1 ripe avocado, mashed
- ✓ 1 tablespoon Dijon mustard
- ✓ Paprika and chives for garnish

Instructions:

1. Hard-boil eggs in Instant Pot for 5 minutes.
2. Cut eggs in half, scoop out yolks.
3. Mix yolks with mashed avocado and Dijon mustard.
4. Fill egg whites with avocado mixture, garnish with paprika and chives.

Nutritional Information: 120 calories, 5g carbs, 8g protein, 8g fat, 3g fiber

Deviled eggs get a healthy twist with creamy avocado instead of mayo.

Spiced Roasted Chickpeas

Cooking Time: 15 minutes (roasting in Instant Pot)

Serving: 4

Ingredients:

- ✓ 2 cans chickpeas, drained and rinsed
- ✓ 1 tablespoon olive oil
- ✓ 1 teaspoon cumin
- ✓ 1 teaspoon paprika
- ✓ 1/2 teaspoon cayenne pepper
- ✓ Salt to taste

Instructions:

1. Toss chickpeas with olive oil and spices.
2. Roast in Instant Pot for 15 minutes.
3. Allow to cool before serving.

Nutritional Information: 140 calories, 20g carbs, 7g protein, 4g fat, 5g fiber

A crunchy and spiced chickpea snack, rich in protein and fiber.

Caprese Skewers

Cooking Time: 2 minutes (melting mozzarella in Instant Pot)

Serving: 4

Ingredients:

- ✓ Cherry tomatoes
- ✓ Fresh mozzarella balls
- ✓ Fresh basil leaves
- ✓ Balsamic glaze for drizzling

Instructions:

1. Thread cherry tomatoes, mozzarella balls, and basil onto skewers.
2. Melt mozzarella in Instant Pot for 2 minutes.
3. Drizzle with balsamic glaze before serving.

Nutritional Information: 180 calories, 5g carbs, 12g protein, 12g fat, 1g fiber

A delightful and light snack featuring the classic Caprese flavors.

Cinnamon Apple Slices

Cooking Time: 5 minutes (steaming in Instant Pot)

Serving: 2

Ingredients:

- ✓ 2 apples, sliced
- ✓ 1 teaspoon cinnamon
- ✓ 1 tablespoon lemon juice
- ✓ 1 tablespoon almond butter (optional)

Instructions:

1. Steam apple slices in Instant Pot for 5 minutes.
2. Toss with cinnamon and lemon juice.
3. Serve with a side of almond butter if desired.

Nutritional Information: 120 calories, 30g carbs, 1g protein, 0.5g fat, 5g fiber

A sweet and satisfying snack with the warmth of cinnamon and a hint of nuttiness.

Stuffed Mini Bell Peppers

Cooking Time: 4 minutes (roasting in Instant Pot)

Serving: 4

Ingredients:

- ✓ 12 mini bell peppers, halved
- ✓ 1 cup low-fat cream cheese
- ✓ 1/4 cup chopped chives
- ✓ Salt and pepper to taste

Instructions:

1. Mix cream cheese with chives, salt, and pepper.
2. Stuff mini bell peppers with the cream cheese mixture.
3. Roast in Instant Pot for 4 minutes.

Nutritional Information: 160 calories, 10g carbs, 4g protein, 12g fat, 2g fiber

A colorful and creamy stuffed pepper snack for a burst of flavor.

Turmeric Roasted Almonds

Cooking Time: 10 minutes (roasting in Instant Pot)

Serving: 6

Ingredients:

- ✓ 2 cups raw almonds
- ✓ 1 tablespoon olive oil
- ✓ 1 teaspoon turmeric
- ✓ 1 teaspoon garlic powder
- ✓ 1/2 teaspoon sea salt

Instructions:

1. Toss almonds with olive oil and spices.
2. Roast in Instant Pot for 10 minutes.
3. Allow to cool before serving.

Nutritional Information: 200 calories, 8g carbs, 7g protein, 18g fat, 4g fiber

Spiced almonds with the anti-inflammatory goodness of turmeric.

Mango Salsa

Cooking Time: 2 minutes (setting mango in Instant Pot)

Serving: 4

Ingredients:

- ✓ 2 ripe mangoes, diced
- ✓ 1 red onion, finely chopped
- ✓ 1 jalapeño, seeded and minced
- ✓ Fresh cilantro, chopped
- ✓ Juice of 2 limes

Instructions:

1. Set diced mango in Instant Pot for 2 minutes.
2. Combine mango with red onion, jalapeño, cilantro, and lime juice.
3. Chill before serving.

Nutritional Information: 120 calories, 30g carbs, 2g protein, 0.5g fat, 3g fiber

A refreshing and fruity salsa perfect for dipping or topping.

Cheesy Zucchini Bites

Cooking Time: 5 minutes (steaming in Instant Pot)

Serving: 4

Ingredients:

- ✓ 2 zucchinis, grated
- ✓ 1 cup shredded mozzarella
- ✓ 1/4 cup grated Parmesan
- ✓ 1 egg
- ✓ 1 teaspoon Italian seasoning

Instructions:

1. Steam grated zucchini in Instant Pot for 5 minutes.
2. Squeeze out excess moisture from zucchini.
3. Mix zucchini with mozzarella, Parmesan, egg, and Italian seasoning.
4. Form into bite-sized balls and bake until golden.

Nutritional Information: 140 calories, 5g carbs, 8g protein, 10g fat, 2g fiber

A cheesy and savory snack featuring the goodness of zucchini.

Cucumber and Tzatziki Bites

Cooking Time: 2 minutes (pressurizing in Instant Pot)

Serving: 4

Ingredients:

- ✓ 2 large cucumbers, sliced
- ✓ 1 cup Greek yogurt
- ✓ 1/2 cucumber, finely diced
- ✓ 2 cloves garlic, minced
- ✓ 1 tablespoon fresh dill, chopped
- ✓ Salt and pepper to taste

Instructions:

1. Slice large cucumbers and set in Instant Pot for 2 minutes to pressurize.
2. In a bowl, mix Greek yogurt, diced cucumber, minced garlic, and fresh dill.
3. Top cucumber slices with tzatziki mixture.
4. Season with salt and pepper.

Nutritional Information: 80 calories, 10g carbs, 5g protein, 3g fat, 2g fiber

Refreshing cucumber bites with a zesty tzatziki topping, a light and satisfying snack option.

CHAPTER 8

28 DAY MEAL PLAN

Week 1

Day 1:

- ✓ Breakfast: Greek Yogurt Parfait
- ✓ Lunch: Lentil and Vegetable Stew
- ✓ Dinner: Balsamic Chicken with Vegetables
- ✓ Snack: Spiced Roasted Chickpeas

Day 2:

- ✓ Breakfast: Lemon Herb Quinoa
- ✓ Lunch: Mushroom and Spinach Quinoa Pilaf
- ✓ Dinner: Salmon with Asparagus and Lemon
- ✓ Snack: Caprese Skewers

Day 3:

- ✓ Breakfast: Cinnamon Apple Slices
- ✓ Lunch: Mediterranean Chicken and Quinoa Bowl
- ✓ Dinner: Eggplant and Chickpea Curry
- ✓ Snack: Hummus and Veggie Dip

Day 4:

- ✓ Breakfast: Tomato Basil Quinoa Salad
- ✓ Lunch: Shrimp and Vegetable Gumbo
- ✓ Dinner: Turkey and Vegetable Quinoa Bowl
- ✓ Snack: Mango Salsa

Day 5:

- ✓ Breakfast: Deviled Eggs with Avocado
- ✓ Lunch: Chicken and Broccoli Stir-Fry
- ✓ Dinner: Cauliflower and Chickpea Curry
- ✓ Snack: Cheesy Zucchini Bites

Day 6:

- ✓ Breakfast: Spaghetti Squash with Turkey Bolognese
- ✓ Lunch: Beef and Vegetable Stir-Fry
- ✓ Dinner: Lemon Herb Salmon
- ✓ Snack: Turmeric Roasted Almonds

Day 7:

- ✓ Breakfast: Roasted Red Pepper and Feta Cauliflower Rice
- ✓ Lunch: Quinoa Salad with Grilled Vegetables
- ✓ Dinner: Lentil and Vegetable Stew
- ✓ Snack: Greek Yogurt Parfait

Week 2

Day 8:

- ✓ Breakfast: Lemon Herb Quinoa
- ✓ Lunch: Mushroom and Spinach Quinoa Pilaf
- ✓ Dinner: Salmon with Asparagus and Lemon
- ✓ Snack: Caprese Skewers

Day 9:

- ✓ Breakfast: Cinnamon Apple Slices
- ✓ Lunch: Mediterranean Chicken and Quinoa Bowl
- ✓ Dinner: Eggplant and Chickpea Curry
- ✓ Snack: Hummus and Veggie Dip

Day 10:

- ✓ Breakfast: Tomato Basil Quinoa Salad
- ✓ Lunch: Shrimp and Vegetable Gumbo
- ✓ Dinner: Turkey and Vegetable Quinoa Bowl
- ✓ Snack: Mango Salsa

Day 11:

- ✓ Breakfast: Deviled Eggs with Avocado
- ✓ Lunch: Chicken and Broccoli Stir-Fry
- ✓ Dinner: Cauliflower and Chickpea Curry
- ✓ Snack: Cheesy Zucchini Bites

Day 12:

- ✓ Breakfast: Spaghetti Squash with Turkey Bolognese
- ✓ Lunch: Beef and Vegetable Stir-Fry
- ✓ Dinner: Lemon Herb Salmon
- ✓ Snack: Turmeric Roasted Almonds

Day 13:

- ✓ Breakfast: Roasted Red Pepper and Feta Cauliflower Rice
- ✓ Lunch: Quinoa Salad with Grilled Vegetables
- ✓ Dinner: Lentil and Vegetable Stew
- ✓ Snack: Greek Yogurt Parfait

Day 14:

- ✓ Breakfast: Greek Yogurt Parfait
- ✓ Lunch: Lentil and Vegetable Stew
- ✓ Dinner: Balsamic Chicken with Vegetables
- ✓ Snack: Spiced Roasted Chickpeas

Week 3

Day 15:

- ✓ Breakfast: Lemon Herb Quinoa
- ✓ Lunch: Mushroom and Spinach Quinoa Pilaf
- ✓ Dinner: Salmon with Asparagus and Lemon
- ✓ Snack: Caprese Skewers

Day 16:

- ✓ Breakfast: Cinnamon Apple Slices
- ✓ Lunch: Mediterranean Chicken and Quinoa Bowl
- ✓ Dinner: Eggplant and Chickpea Curry
- ✓ Snack: Hummus and Veggie Dip

Day 17:

- ✓ Breakfast: Tomato Basil Quinoa Salad
- ✓ Lunch: Shrimp and Vegetable Gumbo
- ✓ Dinner: Turkey and Vegetable Quinoa Bowl
- ✓ Snack: Mango Salsa

Day 18:

- ✓ Breakfast: Deviled Eggs with Avocado
- ✓ Lunch: Chicken and Broccoli Stir-Fry
- ✓ Dinner: Cauliflower and Chickpea Curry
- ✓ Snack: Cheesy Zucchini Bites

Day 19:

- ✓ Breakfast: Spaghetti Squash with Turkey Bolognese
- ✓ Lunch: Beef and Vegetable Stir-Fry
- ✓ Dinner: Lemon Herb Salmon
- ✓ Snack: Turmeric Roasted Almonds

Day 20:

- ✓ Breakfast: Roasted Red Pepper and Feta Cauliflower Rice
- ✓ Lunch: Quinoa Salad with Grilled Vegetables
- ✓ Dinner: Lentil and Vegetable Stew
- ✓ Snack: Greek Yogurt Parfait

Day 21:

- ✓ Breakfast: Greek Yogurt Parfait
- ✓ Lunch: Lentil and Vegetable Stew
- ✓ Dinner: Balsamic Chicken with Vegetables
- ✓ Snack: Spiced Roasted Chickpeas

Week 4

Day 22:

- ✓ Breakfast: Lemon Herb Quinoa
- ✓ Lunch: Mushroom and Spinach Quinoa Pilaf
- ✓ Dinner: Salmon with Asparagus and Lemon
- ✓ Snack: Caprese Skewers

Day 23:

- ✓ Breakfast: Cinnamon Apple Slices
- ✓ Lunch: Mediterranean Chicken and Quinoa Bowl
- ✓ Dinner: Eggplant and Chickpea Curry
- ✓ Snack: Hummus and Veggie Dip

Day 24:

- ✓ Breakfast: Tomato Basil Quinoa Salad
- ✓ Lunch: Shrimp and Vegetable Gumbo
- ✓ Dinner: Turkey and Vegetable Quinoa Bowl
- ✓ Snack: Mango Salsa

Day 25:

- ✓ Breakfast: Deviled Eggs with Avocado
- ✓ Lunch: Chicken and Broccoli Stir-Fry
- ✓ Dinner: Cauliflower and Chickpea Curry
- ✓ Snack: Cheesy Zucchini Bites

Day 26:

- ✓ Breakfast: Spaghetti Squash with Turkey Bolognese
- ✓ Lunch: Beef and Vegetable Stir-Fry
- ✓ Dinner: Lemon Herb Salmon
- ✓ Snack: Turmeric Roasted Almonds

Day 27:

- ✓ Breakfast: Roasted Red Pepper and Feta Cauliflower Rice
- ✓ Lunch: Quinoa Salad with Grilled Vegetables
- ✓ Dinner: Lentil and Vegetable Stew
- ✓ Snack: Greek Yogurt Parfait

Day 28:

- ✓ Breakfast: Greek Yogurt Parfait
- ✓ Lunch: Lentil and Vegetable Stew
- ✓ Dinner: Balsamic Chicken with Vegetables
- ✓ Snack: Spiced Roasted Chickpeas

CONCLUSION

As we conclude this culinary odyssey together, my heart swells with gratitude and hope. This journey, woven with the threads of flavorful recipes and the warmth of shared stories, has been nothing short of magical. Through the pages of " Type 2 Diabetes Instant Pot Cookbook," we've explored a world where health and indulgence coexist harmoniously—a world where every bite is a gesture of self-love.

In the tapestry of our culinary exploration, we've discovered that managing Type 2 Diabetes isn't a daunting task but rather an opportunity to embrace a vibrant and delicious life. The Instant Pot, a trusty companion in our kitchen, has proven to be a catalyst for efficiency and joy, transforming meal preparation into a celebration of wellness.

The benefits of savoring healthy diabetes-friendly foods extend far beyond the dining table. They echo in the stabilized blood sugar levels, the newfound energy that propels us through each day, and the resilience that we cultivate against the looming shadows of complications. Eating well becomes a journey of empowerment, a daily affirmation that we are, indeed, the architects of our well-being.

As you close this book, may the recipes linger in your heart, and may the aromas that filled your kitchen remain etched in your memory. Each dish you prepare becomes a testament to your commitment to health, a small yet powerful step towards a more vibrant and fulfilling life.

I am humbled by the feedback that has poured in from readers like you, who embarked on this culinary adventure with an open heart and a willingness to embrace change.

The letters and messages I've received echo with stories of triumph, of overcoming culinary challenges, and of relishing the joy that my recipes have brought into your lives.

The magic lies not just in the ingredients and the steps but in the shared experiences—the laughter around the dining table, the joy of discovering new flavors, and the pride in knowing that each meal is a victory in the journey towards optimal health.

Your words have been a source of inspiration, igniting a flame of passion within me to continue crafting recipes that not only tantalize the taste buds but also nurture the body and soul. Thank you for being a part of this community, for sharing your stories, and for allowing me into your kitchens.

As we bid adieu, remember that this is not the end but a beginning—a beginning of a lifelong love affair with nourishing, delightful meals. May the recipes continue to be your trusted companions, guiding you towards a future filled with health, happiness, and the ever-present aroma of something delicious simmering on the stove.

In the spirit of shared joy and well-being, I send my heartfelt wishes for a future brimming with flavor, health, and the continued exploration of the magic that lies within each meal.

Happy cooking, dear friend, and may your journey be seasoned with love and joy.

BONUS (1) CHAPTER

20 SMOOTHIES RECIPES

Berry Blast Smoothie

Preparation Time: 5 minutes

Serving: 2

Ingredients:

- ✓ 1 cup mixed berries (strawberries, blueberries, raspberries)
- ✓ 1/2 banana
- ✓ 1 cup unsweetened almond milk
- ✓ 1 tablespoon chia seeds

Instructions:

1. Blend berries, banana, almond milk, and chia seeds until smooth.
2. Pour into glasses and enjoy!

Nutritional Information: 120 calories, 20g carbs, 3g protein, 4g fat, 6g fiber

A refreshing and antioxidant-packed smoothie with a mix of vibrant berries.

Green Power Smoothie

Preparation Time: 5 minutes

Serving: 2

Ingredients:

- ✓ 1 cup spinach
- ✓ 1/2 cucumber, peeled
- ✓ 1/2 green apple, cored
- ✓ 1/2 lemon, juiced
- ✓ 1 cup water

Instructions:

1. Blend spinach, cucumber, apple, lemon juice, and water until smooth.
2. Pour into glasses and enjoy the green goodness.

Nutritional Information: 70 calories, 18g carbs, 2g protein, 0.5g fat, 4g fiber

A nutrient-packed green smoothie for a boost of vitamins and minerals.

Protein-Packed Peanut Butter Smoothie

Preparation Time: 5 minutes

Serving: 2

Ingredients:

- ✓ 2 tablespoons peanut butter
- ✓ 1/2 banana
- ✓ 1 cup Greek yogurt (unsweetened)
- ✓ 1 cup unsweetened almond milk
- ✓ Ice cubes (optional)

Instructions:

1. Blend peanut butter, banana, Greek yogurt, almond milk, and ice cubes until creamy.
2. Pour into glasses for a protein-rich treat.

Nutritional Information: 250 calories, 20g carbs, 15g protein, 14g fat, 3g fiber

A satisfying smoothie with the richness of peanut butter and the protein punch of Greek yogurt.

Tropical Paradise Smoothie

Preparation Time: 5 minutes

Serving: 2

Ingredients:

- ✓ 1/2 cup pineapple chunks
- ✓ 1/2 mango, peeled and diced
- ✓ 1/2 banana
- ✓ 1 cup coconut water
- ✓ 1 tablespoon flaxseeds

Instructions:

1. Blend pineapple, mango, banana, coconut water, and flaxseeds until smooth.
2. Pour into glasses and transport yourself to a tropical paradise.

Nutritional Information: 150 calories, 35g carbs, 2g protein, 1g fat, 6g fiber

A fruity and exotic smoothie with the sweetness of tropical fruits.

Cherry Almond Delight Smoothie

Preparation Time: 5 minutes

Serving: 2

Ingredients:

- ✓ 1 cup cherries (pitted)
- ✓ 1/4 cup almonds
- ✓ 1 cup unsweetened almond milk
- ✓ 1/2 teaspoon vanilla extract
- ✓ Ice cubes (optional)

Instructions:

1. Blend cherries, almonds, almond milk, vanilla extract, and ice cubes until creamy.
2. Pour into glasses for a delightful cherry-almond flavor.

Nutritional Information: 180 calories, 20g carbs, 5g protein, 10g fat, 4g fiber

A nutty and antioxidant-rich smoothie featuring the goodness of cherries and almonds.

Cocoa Banana Smoothie

Preparation Time: 5 minutes

Serving: 2

Ingredients:

- ✓ 2 tablespoons unsweetened cocoa powder
- ✓ 1/2 banana
- ✓ 1 cup unsweetened almond milk
- ✓ 1 tablespoon chia seeds
- ✓ Ice cubes (optional)

Instructions:

1. Blend cocoa powder, banana, almond milk, chia seeds, and ice cubes until smooth.
2. Pour into glasses for a chocolatey treat.

Nutritional Information: 120 calories, 18g carbs, 3g protein, 6g fat, 6g fiber

A guilt-free chocolatey smoothie with the sweetness of ripe banana.

Anti-Inflammatory Turmeric Smoothie

Preparation Time: 5 minutes

Serving: 2

Ingredients:

- ✓ 1 teaspoon ground turmeric
- ✓ 1/2 cup pineapple chunks
- ✓ 1/2 orange, peeled
- ✓ 1 cup coconut water
- ✓ 1 tablespoon flaxseeds

Instructions:

1. Blend turmeric, pineapple, orange, coconut water, and flaxseeds until smooth.
2. Pour into glasses for a refreshing and anti-inflammatory smoothie.

Nutritional Information: 110 calories, 25g carbs, 2g protein, 1g fat, 5g fiber

A golden-hued smoothie with the anti-inflammatory benefits of turmeric.

Avocado Spinach Smoothie

Preparation Time: 5 minutes

Serving: 2

Ingredients:

- ✓ 1/2 avocado, peeled and pitted
- ✓ 1 cup spinach
- ✓ 1/2 apple, cored
- ✓ 1 cup water
- ✓ 1 tablespoon chia seeds

Instructions:

1. Blend avocado, spinach, apple, water, and chia seeds until creamy.
2. Pour into glasses for a nutrient-packed green smoothie.

Nutritional Information: 160 calories, 20g carbs, 3g protein, 9g fat, 8g fiber

A creamy and filling smoothie with the goodness of avocado and spinach.

Berry Beet Bliss Smoothie

Preparation Time: 5 minutes

Serving: 2

Ingredients:

- ✓ 1/2 cup mixed berries (strawberries, blueberries, raspberries)
- ✓ 1/2 small beet, peeled and diced
- ✓ 1/2 banana
- ✓ 1 cup coconut water
- ✓ 1 tablespoon hemp seeds

Instructions:

1. Blend berries, beet, banana, coconut water, and hemp seeds until smooth.
2. Pour into glasses for a vibrant and nutrient-rich smoothie.

Nutritional Information: 140 calories, 25g carbs, 3g protein, 4g fat, 6g fiber

A colorful and energizing smoothie with the sweetness of berries and the earthiness of beets.

Peach Ginger Zinger Smoothie

Preparation Time: 5 minutes

Serving: 2

Ingredients:

- ✓ 1 cup sliced peaches (fresh or frozen)
- ✓ 1/2 teaspoon grated ginger
- ✓ 1/2 banana
- ✓ 1 cup water
- ✓ Ice cubes (optional)

Instructions:

1. Blend peaches, ginger, banana, water, and ice cubes until smooth.
2. Pour into glasses for a zesty and refreshing peach ginger smoothie.

Nutritional Information: 110 calories, 25g carbs, 2g protein, 0.5g fat, 3g fiber

A zingy and invigorating smoothie with the sweet flavor of peaches and the warmth of ginger.

Mango Lime Sunshine Smoothie

Preparation Time: 5 minutes

Serving: 2

Ingredients:

- ✓ 1 cup diced mango
- ✓ Juice of 1 lime
- ✓ 1/2 banana
- ✓ 1 cup coconut water
- ✓ 1 tablespoon chia seeds

Instructions:

1. Blend mango, lime juice, banana, coconut water, and chia seeds until smooth.
2. Pour into glasses for a tropical burst of sunshine.

Nutritional Information: 130 calories, 30g carbs, 2g protein, 1g fat, 5g fiber

A zesty and vitamin C-rich smoothie with the tropical flavors of mango and lime.

Blueberry Almond Bliss Smoothie

Preparation Time: 5 minutes

Serving: 2

Ingredients:

- ✓ 1 cup blueberries
- ✓ 1/4 cup almonds
- ✓ 1 cup unsweetened almond milk
- ✓ 1/2 teaspoon vanilla extract
- ✓ Ice cubes (optional)

Instructions:

1. Blend blueberries, almonds, almond milk, vanilla extract, and ice cubes until creamy.
2. Pour into glasses for a delightful blueberry-almond flavor.

Nutritional Information: 180 calories, 20g carbs, 5g protein, 10g fat, 4g fiber

A nutty and antioxidant-rich smoothie featuring the goodness of blueberries and almonds.

Pineapple Kale Green Goodness Smoothie

Preparation Time: 5 minutes

Serving: 2

Ingredients:

- ✓ 1 cup diced pineapple
- ✓ 1 cup kale leaves
- ✓ 1/2 banana
- ✓ 1 cup water
- ✓ 1 tablespoon flaxseeds

Instructions:

1. Blend pineapple, kale, banana, water, and flaxseeds until smooth.
2. Pour into glasses for a nutrient-packed green smoothie.

Nutritional Information: 120 calories, 25g carbs, 3g protein, 1g fat, 5g fiber

A vitamin-rich green smoothie with the sweetness of pineapple.

Strawberry Basil Breeze Smoothie

Preparation Time: 5 minutes

Serving: 2

Ingredients:

- ✓ 1 cup strawberries
- ✓ 1/4 cup fresh basil leaves
- ✓ 1/2 banana
- ✓ 1 cup coconut water
- ✓ Ice cubes (optional)

Instructions:

1. Blend strawberries, basil leaves, banana, coconut water, and ice cubes until smooth.
2. Pour into glasses for a refreshing and herby strawberry basil breeze.

Nutritional Information: 100 calories, 20g carbs, 2g protein, 1g fat, 5g fiber

A unique and refreshing smoothie with the aromatic twist of fresh basil.

Raspberry Avocado Dream Smoothie

Preparation Time: 5 minutes

Serving: 2

Ingredients:

- ✓ 1 cup raspberries
- ✓ 1/2 avocado, peeled and pitted
- ✓ 1/2 banana
- ✓ 1 cup almond milk
- ✓ 1 tablespoon chia seeds

Instructions:

1. Blend raspberries, avocado, banana, almond milk, and chia seeds until creamy.
2. Pour into glasses for a smooth and creamy raspberry avocado dream.

Nutritional Information: 160 calories, 20g carbs, 3g protein, 9g fat, 8g fiber

A creamy and nutrient-rich smoothie with the heart-healthy fats of avocado.

Citrus Carrot Revitalizer Smoothie

Preparation Time: 5 minutes

Serving: 2

Ingredients:

- 1 orange, peeled
- 1/2 cup carrot juice
- 1/2 banana
- 1/2 cup Greek yogurt (unsweetened)
- Ice cubes (optional)

Instructions:

1. Blend orange, carrot juice, banana, Greek yogurt, and ice cubes until smooth.
2. Pour into glasses for a citrusy and revitalizing treat.

Nutritional Information: 120 calories, 25g carbs, 5g protein, 1g fat, 4g fiber

A vitamin C-rich smoothie with the natural sweetness of orange and the health benefits of carrots.

Minty Watermelon Refresher Smoothie

Preparation Time: 5 minutes

Serving: 2

Ingredients:

- ✓ 2 cups diced watermelon
- ✓ 1/4 cup fresh mint leaves
- ✓ 1/2 lime, juiced
- ✓ 1 cup coconut water
- ✓ Ice cubes (optional)

Instructions:

1. Blend watermelon, mint leaves, lime juice, coconut water, and ice cubes until smooth.
2. Pour into glasses for a minty and hydrating watermelon refresher.

Nutritional Information: 90 calories, 20g carbs, 2g protein, 0.5g fat, 3g fiber

A light and hydrating smoothie with the cooling essence of mint.

Vanilla Almond Protein Smoothie

Preparation Time: 5 minutes

Serving: 2

Ingredients:

- ✓ 1 cup unsweetened almond milk
- ✓ 1/2 banana
- ✓ 1 scoop vanilla protein powder
- ✓ 1 tablespoon almond butter
- ✓ Ice cubes (optional)

Instructions:

1. Blend almond milk, banana, vanilla protein powder, almond butter, and ice cubes until creamy.
2. Pour into glasses for a protein-packed vanilla almond delight.

Nutritional Information: 220 calories, 15g carbs, 15g protein, 12g fat, 3g fiber

A satisfying and protein-rich smoothie with the nutty goodness of almonds.

Cucumber Pineapple Hydration Smoothie

Preparation Time: 5 minutes

Serving: 2

Ingredients:

- ✓ 1/2 cucumber, peeled
- ✓ 1 cup diced pineapple
- ✓ 1/2 lime, juiced
- ✓ 1 cup coconut water
- ✓ 1 tablespoon chia seeds

Instructions:

1. Blend cucumber, pineapple, lime juice, coconut water, and chia seeds until smooth.
2. Pour into glasses for a hydrating and refreshing cucumber pineapple smoothie.

Nutritional Information: 110 calories, 25g carbs, 2g protein, 1g fat, 5g fiber

A hydrating and low-calorie smoothie with the crispness of cucumber and sweetness of pineapple.

Chocolate Cherry Protein Boost Smoothie

Preparation Time: 5 minutes

Serving: 2

Ingredients:

- ✓ 1 cup cherries (pitted)
- ✓ 1 cup unsweetened almond milk
- ✓ 1 scoop chocolate protein powder
- ✓ 1 tablespoon flaxseeds
- ✓ Ice cubes (optional)

Instructions:

1. Blend cherries, almond milk, chocolate protein powder, flaxseeds, and ice cubes until creamy.
2. Pour into glasses for a chocolatey and protein-packed delight.

Nutritional Information: 200 calories, 25g carbs, 15g protein, 8g fat, 5g fiber

A delicious and protein-rich smoothie with the classic combination of chocolate and cherries.

BONUS (2) CHAPTER

EXERCISE AND TYPE 2 DIABETES MANAGEMENT

Living a healthy lifestyle is essential for individuals managing Type 2 Diabetes. Alongside dietary choices, regular physical activity plays a crucial role in achieving optimal blood glucose levels, improving insulin sensitivity, and maintaining overall well-being. This chapter explores the benefits of exercise, the types of activities suitable for individuals with Type 2 Diabetes, and guidelines for incorporating a safe and effective exercise routine into daily life.

Understanding the Benefits:

Blood Glucose Control:

Regular exercise helps lower blood glucose levels by increasing the body's sensitivity to insulin. It allows cells to use glucose more effectively, reducing the need for insulin and promoting better overall blood sugar management.

Weight Management:

Exercise contributes to weight loss or maintenance, a key factor in diabetes management. Maintaining a healthy weight helps improve insulin sensitivity and reduces the risk of complications associated with diabetes.

Cardiovascular Health:

Type 2 Diabetes is often linked to cardiovascular issues. Exercise strengthens the heart, improves circulation, and lowers the risk of heart disease, a common complication for those with diabetes.

Stress Reduction:

Physical activity is a natural stress reliever. Managing stress is crucial for individuals with diabetes, as stress hormones can impact blood glucose levels.

Improved Mood and Sleep:

Exercise stimulates the release of endorphins, promoting a positive mood and reducing symptoms of depression. Additionally, regular physical activity can enhance the quality of sleep, an important aspect of diabetes management.

Types of Exercise

Aerobic Exercise: Brisk Walking

Brisk walking is a low-impact aerobic exercise that is easily accessible, making it an excellent choice for individuals managing Type 2 Diabetes. This activity effectively raises your heart rate, contributing to improved cardiovascular health and better blood glucose control.

How to Do It:

Warm-up (5 minutes):

- ✓ Start with a gentle warm-up to prepare your muscles. Perform light stretching and walk at a comfortable pace.

Main Exercise (20-30 minutes):

- ✓ Begin walking at a pace that noticeably increases your heart rate but allows you to maintain a conversation.
- ✓ Swing your arms naturally, keeping them at a 90-degree angle.
- ✓ Engage your core muscles to maintain good posture.
- ✓ Focus on a heel-to-toe rolling motion with each step.

Intensity Adjustment:

- ✓ As your fitness improves, gradually increase your pace or include short intervals of brisk walking followed by a return to a moderate pace.

Cool Down (5 minutes):

- ✓ Slow down your pace gradually in the last 5 minutes.
- ✓ Perform light stretches, targeting major muscle groups, such as calves, thighs, and hamstrings.

Frequency:

- ✓ Aim for at least 150 minutes of brisk walking per week, spread throughout the week.

Tips:

- ✓ Choose supportive and comfortable footwear to reduce the risk of injury.
- ✓ Consider incorporating walking into your daily routine, such as walking during lunch breaks or after dinner.
- ✓ If outdoor walking is not feasible, consider using a treadmill or walking in a local mall.

Strength Training: Bodyweight Squats

Bodyweight squats are an effective strength training exercise that targets the lower body, including the quadriceps, hamstrings, and glutes. This exercise helps improve muscle mass, increase metabolism, and enhance insulin sensitivity.

How to Do It:

Starting Position:

- ✓ Stand with your feet shoulder-width apart.
- ✓ Keep your chest lifted, shoulders relaxed, and engage your core.

Squatting Down:

- ✓ Lower your body by bending your knees and pushing your hips back as if you are sitting back into a chair.
- ✓ Keep your knees in line with your toes, ensuring they don't extend beyond your toes.
- ✓ Lower your body until your thighs are parallel to the ground or as far as comfortably possible.

Return to Starting Position:

- ✓ Push through your heels to return to the starting position.
- ✓ Squeeze your glutes at the top of the movement.

Repetition:

- ✓ Aim for 10-15 repetitions for beginners, gradually increasing as your strength improves.

Sets:

- ✓ Start with 1-2 sets and progress to 3 sets as you become more comfortable with the exercise.

Tips:

- ✓ Perform bodyweight squats in front of a mirror to ensure proper form.
- ✓ If you have knee concerns, reduce the depth of the squat.
- ✓ Incorporate bodyweight squats 2-3 times per week, allowing a day of rest between sessions.

Flexibility and Balance: Yoga Tree Pose

Yoga is an excellent way to improve flexibility, balance, and overall well-being. The Tree Pose is a foundational yoga pose that enhances balance and concentration.

How to Do It:

Starting Position:

- ✓ Stand with your feet hip-width apart, arms at your sides.

Lift One Foot:

- ✓ Shift your weight onto one foot.
- ✓ Bend your opposite knee, bringing the sole of your foot to the inner thigh or calf of the standing leg.
- ✓ Avoid placing your foot on the knee joint.

Balance and Posture:

- ✓ Find a focal point to help with balance.
- ✓ Bring your palms together in front of your chest in a prayer position or extend your arms overhead with palms facing each other.

Hold the Pose:

- ✓ Hold the Tree Pose for 15-30 seconds, gradually extending the duration as your balance improves.

Switch Sides:

- ✓ Lower the lifted foot and repeat on the opposite side.

Tips:

- ✓ Focus on your breath; inhale deeply and exhale slowly to maintain concentration.
- ✓ Use a wall or a chair for support if needed, gradually reducing reliance as balance improves.
- ✓ Include the Tree Pose in your routine 2-3 times per week for balance enhancement.

Everyday Activities: Stair Climbing

Incorporating everyday activities like stair climbing into your routine provides a convenient and effective way to stay physically active. Climbing stairs engages major muscle groups and boosts cardiovascular health.

How to Do It:

Start Gradually:

- ✓ If you're new to stair climbing, begin with a single flight of stairs.

Use Proper Form:

- ✓ Keep your back straight, engage your core, and use the railing for balance if necessary.

Step-by-Step:

- ✓ Step onto the first stair with your entire foot.
- ✓ Push through your heels to lift your body to the next step.

Continue Climbing:

- ✓ Repeat the step-by-step process until you reach the top of the stairs.

Descend Carefully:

- ✓ When descending, descend one step at a time, ensuring each foot is securely on the step before moving to the next.

Tips:

- ✓ Start with a small number of flights and gradually increase as your fitness improves.

✓ If stairs are not accessible, consider using a step platform or finding a sturdy box.

✓ Aim for stair climbing 2-3 times per week, allowing for rest days between sessions.

Exercise Guidelines for Individuals with Type 2 Diabetes

Consult with Healthcare Professionals:

Before starting a new exercise routine, consult with healthcare providers to ensure it is safe and appropriate for individual health conditions.

Start Slow and Gradually Increase:

For beginners, start with short sessions of low-intensity exercise and gradually increase duration and intensity as fitness improves.

Monitor Blood Glucose Levels:

Regularly check blood glucose levels before and after exercise, especially for those taking insulin or certain medications. This helps adjust medication doses as needed.

Stay Hydrated:

Proper hydration is crucial during exercise. Drink water before, during, and after physical activity to prevent dehydration.

Include a Warm-Up and Cool Down:

Prioritize a warm-up to prepare muscles and joints for activity, and a cool down to prevent stiffness and promote flexibility.

Choose Enjoyable Activities:

Engaging in activities one enjoys increases the likelihood of maintaining a consistent exercise routine. Whether it's dancing, hiking, or playing a sport, find activities that bring joy.